Homemade Hand Sanitizer

A practical and easy guide to make your own homemade hand sanitizer to protect yourself from germs

Copyright © 2020 Eugene Jenner

All rights reserved.

It is not legal to reproduce, duplicate, or transmit any part of this document by either electronic means or in printed format. Recording of this publication is strictly prohibited.

Disclaimer

The information in this book is based on personal experience and anecdotal evidence. Although the author has made every attempt to achieve an accuracy of the information gathered in this book, they make no representation or warranties concerning the accuracy or completeness of the contents of this book. Your circumstances may not be suited to some illustrations in this book.

The author disclaims any liability arising directly or indirectly from the use of this book. Readers are encouraged to seek medical accounting, legal or professional help when required.

This guide is for informational purposes only, and the author does not accept any responsability for any liability resulting from the use of this information. While every attempt has been made to verfy the information provided here, the author cannot assume any responsability for errors, inaccuracies or omission.

Table of Contents

Chapter 1: Take Care of your Hands 8
- A Brief History: 9
- How are diseases spread? 11
- What diseases can you prevent? 12
- What kind of germs are present on the hands? 14
- Is water enough to wash your hands? 14
- What are the steps of handwashing? 15
- When should you wash your hands? 17
- Hand Sanitizer: 18
- How to properly use hand sanitizer: 19
- How does it work? 20
- Handwashing vs hand sanitizer: which is better? 20

Chapter 2: Hand Sanitizer 22
- The truth about hand sanitizer: 22
- Dangers of commercial hand sanitizer: 24
- Types of hand sanitizer: 27

Chapter 3: Make your own Hand Sanitizer 29
- Hand sanitizers in healthcare setting: 30
- Alcoholic hand sanitizer recipes 39
- Non-Alcoholic hand sanitizer recipes 45

- Hand sanitizer for kids: 60

Chapter 4:Safety Consideration.. 66
- How to prevent yourself from getting sick:............. 67

Introduction

It's the year 2020 as the world heads towards yet another pandemic. This time it"s called Covid 2019 that is wreaking havoc all across the world, spreading like wildfire. It moves from one continent to another, one country to the next as we hold our breath and wait for it to somehow skip us.

Covid-19 is a disease caused by Severe acute respiratory syndrome coronavirus 2 (SARS-CoV-2) and it first started to spread in China. While in majority of cases only mild symptoms are produced, it can also be fatal in a very small percentage of people. Like common cold or flu, coronavirus is also spreads through respiratory droplets. But what is it that makes this disease spread so fast? And what is it that we can do to ensure that we save ourselves from it? A simple technique: Handwashing.

Handwashing is the key to saving yourself from getting affected by this mysterious disease and many other contagious diseases. But it's not just a simple wash with water, you need to learn the proper technique of handwashing as outlined by WHO as well as know what else you can use to keep your hands clean at all times. Knowing that it is not possible or practical to wash hands again and again, a hand sanitizer is what keeps you safe from this virus when you are outside. But hand sanitizers are expensive and exactly how many hand sanitizers are you going to buy? And for how long? This book provides a quick guide to solve all of these problems and answer all of these questions.

Hand hygiene is important in keeping yourself safe from not only coronaviruses but many other diseases too. This includes stomach bugs, cholera, and different varieties of flu. To maintain hand hygiene, it is important to observe proper handwashing as well as use hand sanitizers when water is not accessible.

In this book, we discuss how important hand hygiene is to keep yourself safe from viruses and bacteria. As we go along, we also explore how you can make your own hand sanitizer, wipes or liquid soaps at home and avoid unnecessary trips to super markets trying to find the right product. You will also get to know about the main constituents of hand sanitizers and the uses of each. It is also very important to differentiate facts from myths. And since there have been many myths regarding hand sanitizers going around, we deemed it necessary to pay some attention towards this aspect too. Therefore, we have also included myth busters about hand sanitizers that are sure to help you understand it better.

I hope you find this text not only informative, but enjoyable as well.

Chapter 1:

Take Care of your Hands

How many things did your hands touch an hour after you woke up this morning? From holding the side of the bed, to turning the door knob, to checking your mobile phone, to your own face, the list goes on. If you start counting the number of places your hands have been in hours after you start a new day, you'll be amazed. Our hands are literally carriers of thousands of microbes that we gather all day from everything we touch. If you google images of culturing bacteria from hands, you'll think a lot before putting your hand on your face. You will rush to wash your hands after getting them dirty in the mud, but will probably not give a second thought after coming back with clean hands from a grocery store.

That's the thing. Because we cannot see these tiny germs, we don't really go and wash our hands until we see something visible. And that is also the advantage that these microorganisms get in spreading from one person to next. According to estimates by Centres of Disease Control (CDC), upto 80% of all infections are spread via hands. Taking care of your hands is an extremely important step in preventing the spread of countless diseases. Just using soap and water, or a sanitizer can help you from contracting various bacterial or viral illnesses.

A Brief History:

Hand hygiene, or hand washing, is the way of using water and/or chemicals to remove dirt, bacteria or viruses from your hands. Handwashing has been a measure of hygiene for as far back as we can see. Many religions also promote handwashing rituals. Interestingly, up until a few decades ago, we did not know what it was that actually caused disease and how handwashing could revolutionize the prevention and limit the spread of diseases. The history of handwashing is quite interesting to note.

Ignaz Phillip Semmelweis, the father of hand hygiene, was a Hungarian physicist and scientist born in the year 1818. He worked at Vienna General Hospital in Austria and was also known as the saviour of mothers. He worked at this hospital, examining patients every morning before rounds, assisting his seniors and helping with deliveries. There were two maternity clinics at the hospital but something very strange was observed. One of these clinics had a very high mortality rate when compared to another. This observation intrigued Semmelweis who saw women begging to get admitted to the clinic with lower mortality rate, even though both clinics practiced the same methods. Semmelweis started to point out all the differences between the two clinics and found none other than the people working at these clinics: one had medical students while the other had midwives.

In 1847, when his friend died, with the same pathology as those women at the clinic, after accidentally getting a cut by another student's scalpel while working on a cadaver. He developed a theory saying that these 'cadaverous particles' were the reason of higher mortality as medical students often went to the maternity clinic after practicing on cadavers. He also imposed mandatory handwashing practice with chlorinated lime before examining the patients and this led to tremendous decrease in mortality. Even though his practices were not followed widely but this was a start. Years later, Florence Nightingale also tried to promote hand washing practices by showing how it reduced infections in the hospitals. It was years and years later though, when this was taken seriously and handwashing made mandatory.

A pioneer in antiseptic procedures, Semmelweis, and later Louis Pasteur, who developed the germ theory of disease were able to figure out how disease spreads via microorganisms. And for us to find out how to stop its spread or limit it by maintaining hand hygiene.

How are diseases spread?

Communicable diseases are easily spread by improper hygiene. A single gram of poop can contain about a trillion bacteria or viruses in it that can stay on your hands if you don't wash them after using the toilet or simply changing a baby's diaper. Hundreds of surfaces that we touch all the time might be sneezed or coughed on by other people and contain these germs that we carry in our hands all the time.

Even your mobile phone is a carrier of so many of these germs that you have no idea of. Since we check our phones multiple times during the day, we transfer a lot of germs to our phones. In a recent research, it was found that more than 17,000 bacterial gene copies were present on the surface of mobile phones of teenage students. Another research has found that on average the mobile phones are ten times dirtier than a toilet seat! A soft microfiber cloth can be used to wipe the phone and get rid of many of these microbes. When you touch your face, eat food or rub your nose, these germs, if not washed or cleaned, get an entry into your body. Now these will either make you sick, or sit in your body for some time ready to jump into another person as soon as you contaminate other surfaces that are later touched by other people. In this way, even one person with a communicable disease can put thousands in danger.

Covid-19 is a pandemic because of it being so highly communicable that it takes no time for it to pass from one person to the next. If we limit the spread of these diseases, we can help in fighting against them. By slowing down the spread, we can also gather enough time to not overly burden the healthcare systems.

What diseases can you prevent?

Hand hygiene has long been seen to prevent communicable diseases. There is a long list of diseases that can be prevented with this simple practice. We are sharing a few of these diseases:

1. Covid-19: A novel form of Corona virus, COVID-19 has been declared a pandemic by WHO. Even though the world is still trying to ascertain how deadly the disease is, there is one thing for certain that the scientists know: Washing your hands can limit its destruction

2. Influenza: A simple flu can be deadly for so many people. According to CDC, in the U.S. alone, the flu has caused more than 30 million illnesses, 350,000 hospitalizations and 20 thousand deaths in one season. Apart from getting a flu shot, handwashing can greatly help with this virus.

3. Conjunctivitis: You know all the members of your house might get infected if you wake up in the morning with a pink eye. As your ub those itchy eyes and unknowingly use the same hand to touch everything else in the house, you leave the germs everywhere for anyone else to catch. It is important to use proper handwashing techniques to prevent yourself from contracting this.

4. Typhoid: Salmonella is another bacteria that is easily spread through feco-oral route. You can easily get it if you don't wash your hands after handling raw meat or after using the toilet.

5. Cholera: Another pandemic, cholera, affects an estimated 5 million people worldwide and causes more than 100 thousand deaths a year. Poor sanitation, improper hand hygiene can result in outbreaks of cholera in developing countries.

What kind of germs are present on the hands?

When talking about germs that are usually present on the hands, it is useful to categorize them into two categories: resident microorganisms and transient microorganisms.

Resident flora are the microorganisms present in the superficial layers of the skin. These are present on the skin for protective functions.

Transient flora, on the other hand, are acquired by direct contact with other surfaces that might be contaminated. These transient organisms can then be transferred to other people with contact or enter the body through mucous membranes. These are the organisms that have the potential to cause illnesses.

Is water enough to wash your hands?

Washing your hands with water is obviously better than not washing it altogether. It is, however, important to use a soap or any other cleaner to rid your hands of the germs that you cannot see with naked eye.

You may ask, what do soap and water do? Well, soap and water do not kill the microorganisms but instead they mechanically remove these germs from your hands. A soap acts as a natural surfactant, a quality that makes it a valuable cleanser.

To know that handwashing can help you immensely is not enough, you also need to know the proper technique of handwashing to maximise the benefits.

What are the steps of handwashing?

According to the CDC, washing your hands and drying them properly takes about 2 minutes. It is equal to the time it takes for you to sing a happy birthday song twice. Since we never time ourselves while washing hands, there is a very high probability that we are not taking enough time to wash our hands. So the next time you go to wash your hands, practice this simple technique to make yourself habitual of washing your hands the right way.

There are a few easy steps that should be followed:

1. First of all, open the tap and wet your hands with sufficient water.

2. Now apply a palmful of product, enough to cover both your hands.

3. Rub your hands from palm to palm as you rub

them together to produce some heat when they're cold

4. Put the palm of your right hand over the back of your left hand and interlace your fingers so as to clean between them. Now, put the palm of your left hand over the back of your right hand with interlacing fingers.

5. Again rub your hands palm to palm, but this time interlace your fingers too

6. With interlocked fingers, rub the back of your right hand's fingers on your left palm. Repeat the step with the other hand.

7. Hold your left thumb with your right hand, (the way a child holds it) and do rotational rubbing with your right palm. Repeat this for your other thumb.

8. Now, rinse your hands with water to get rid of the soap

9. Dry your hands thoroughly with a hand towel

10. Use the towel to turn off the faucet before throwing it away (A very important step that

people tend to miss)

11. Once dry, your hands are safe!

These are the steps that should be followed when the hands are visibly dirty or soiled. If you don't see anything on your hands, it does not mean that they are clean. There can be thousands of germs present on the hands that are not visible and so handwashing might be take for granted. Routinely, when hands are visibly clean, you can use a hand sanitizer to practice hand hygiene.

When should you wash your hands?

It is important to keep your hands clean at all times. There are, however, certain occasions when you must ensure that you are washing your hands to keep yourself and others around you healthy.

Some of the times that you must wash your hands are:

1. After using the toilet: To control the spread of diseases that are spread through feco-oral route, it is absolutely essential that you wash your hands after using the toilet. You don't want tiny bits of faeces going into your mouth when you eat, right?

2. Before eating food

3. After touching garbage (that's a no-brainer)

4. Before and after tending to a sick person: You don't want the germs on your hands reaching a person with low immunity and you wouldn't want to catch someone else's communicable disease either.

5. After contact with any other bodily fluids

6. After coming from super markets, playgrounds, public parks or malls

Hand Sanitizer:

A hand sanitizer, simply called a sanitizer, is a disinfectant in the form of a liquid, foam or a gel that is used to remove the unwanted microbes on your skin. If soap and water are not easily accessible, hand sanitizers can be used to keep the hands germ-free.

Hand sanitizers are mostly made up of alcohol. In different types of sanitizers, the amount of alcohol, mentioned as a percentage, varies. Normally a sanitizer is made up of alcohol and water. There are non alcohol based sanitizers too that have not proved to be very useful. We discuss more about the constitution of hand sanitizers in the following chapter.

We have already discussed how it is important to know the proper technique of maintaining hand hygiene to maximise benefits. Now we will see the correct method of using hand sanitizer to make sure that we are following the guidelines.

How to properly use hand sanitizer:

1. Make sure that you do not have any visible dirt on your hands before using the sanitizer

2. Put enough product on your hand to cover the surface of both your hands. Usually, a dime sized amount on your palm is enough

3. Rub your hands together covering your palms, back of your hand and fingers

4. Rub until your hands feel dry. This should take around 15-20 seconds. Make sure that you do not wipe your hands off before the product has dried off.

How does it work?

A hand sanitizer contains alcohol as the main disinfectant. Products that contain at least 60% alcohol work by killing a wide variety of bacteria, including some antibiotic resistant bacteria. It works by destroying the cell surface membranes or enzymes in bacteria, essentially killing them or stopping them from reproducing. It is also true, however, that hand sanitizer cannot kill all kinds of bacteria or viruses. Certain bacteria, like E. Coli, for example, have a thin cell wall that can get easily dissolved in the alcohol and thus makes them susceptible.

Handwashing vs hand sanitizer: which is better?

For routine hygienic antisepsis of your hands, a hand sanitizer is sometimes required. It is a faster way of ensuring that your hands remain clean and you are not spreading any germs around.

Still, apart from healthcare setting, experts recommend maintaining proper hand hygiene by first using the water and soap combination, since there are many germs that might not get killed by a sanitizer. Also, in cases of visible dirt, hand washing is more important.

Chapter 2:

Hand Sanitizer

In this chapter, we are going to look in detail about what hand sanitizers are, how they are made and what are the different types of hand sanitizers that are available commercially.

The truth about hand sanitizer:

As the pandemic coronavirus spreads across the world, we see how countries are facing the crisis. The demand for hand sanitizers jumped up rapidly everywhere and also led to a shortage of these products worldwide. All the spotlight that hand sanitizers are getting is also leading towards some myths being spread. We will try to debunk some of these myths as we go along with this chapter.

Myth 1: Hand sanitizers are a substitute for handwashing.

Answer: Flase. Hand sanitizers can never substitute handwashing. Handwashing still remains the number one line of protection against microbes that get on hands. Using soap and water, as simple as it may sound, still proves to be the most effective against germs.

Myth 2: Hand sanitizers cause antibiotic resistance

Answer: Flase. There isn't sufficient evidence to prove that hand sanitizers cause antibiotic resistance. These products are applied on the skin only and kill the bacteria present there.

Myth 3: All hand sanitizers can work against germs, the composition does not matter

Answer: Flase. Commercially available hand sanitizers have different compositions and all hand sanitizers are not equal in effectiveness. It is essential that you check the composition before buying. According to health experts, for viruses like coronavirus, Covid-19, hand sanitizers must contain at least 60% alcohol to be effective.

Myth 4: Hand sanitizers kill 99.9% germs

Answer: Flase. Hand sanitizers are effective against a wide variety of microorganisms but there is no evidence yet to prove that it kills 99.9% of the germs. Research so far has shown it to be around 60% effective.

Myth 5: A drop or two of hand sanitizer is enough

Answer: False. It is important that you apply enough quantity of hand sanitizer on your hands that you can rub your hands together completely without it drying off.

Myth 6: All alcohol based hand sanitizers contain triclosan

Answer: False. This is a very common myth that has been debunked at a lot of places but people still continue to believe it. Good alcohol based sanitizers, like Purell, do not contain triclosan as one of the ingredients.

Now that we have debunked some myths regarding hand sanitizers, let's go on to talk about how hand sanitizers that are commercially available can pose dangers.

Dangers of commercial hand sanitizer:

First and foremost, let's talk about the use of commercially available hand sanitizers in children. It is tempting to use alcohol based sanitizers to decontaminate surfaces and some people use these products, not just on their hands but on the hands of their kids too. Even the CDC have reported the use of these alcoholic hand sanitizers in children and the risks it poses on their health. The most common adverse effects include irritation of the skin, eye problems or vomiting.

For these reasons, it is suggested to not use these hand sanitizers, particularly with kids 12 years or younger.

However, you do not need to worry. We have a solution for this problem provided in this very book. As you go along the chapters, you will find recipes that contain all natural products that tend to have very few side effects, almost equal to none, and are less likely to cause irritation. We also have provided a special recipe of hand sanitizer that can be used particularly for children.

Another common problem that people face while using some (not all) commercial hand sanitizers is the use of triclosan. Let's discuss a bit about triclosan, what it actually is and why it is sometimes considered harmful.

Triclosan:

Triclosan is an antibacterial and antifungal chemical also called TCS. It is present in many common household products like toothpastes, soaps or detergents. As we have previously discussed, some companies use triclosan in their hand sanitizers too. Even though the use of triclosan in antiseptic washes was prohibited by FDA, it is still sometimes used in some products, and widely used in many other countries too. The ban by FDA in 2016 was due to the fact that there wasn't enough evidence to prove that it was safe to use. Still, the research regarding triclosan is inconclusive and it cannot be said with complete confidence that triclosan is as harmful as it is claimed to be. Many experiments have been conducted on mice to check the effect of triclosan. It was seen to cause inflammation in the gut and later studies have also provided evidence to show that it produces high levels of antibiotic resistant species in the gut.

Triclosan has been a subject of great controversy for a very long time. Even though considered as an antibacterial, the use of triclosan in topical medicines has been discouraged by many health care professionals. Some say that its excessive use can lead to alterations in immunity or cause hormonal problems. However, this is not confirmed yet.

To tackle this issue, it is important to look at the composition of hand sanitizers and see if they are triclosan based.

Many commercially available hand sanitizers contain thousands of chemicals in the name of fragrances. Since there is a great demand for nicely scented products, it is tempting to produce hand sanitizers that smell nice even if that means adding artificial products in it, some scented hand sanitizers can also cause massive irritation on sensitive skin. It can lead to respiratory problems, eczema and other associated issues that can prove to be dangerous with excessive use. Diseases like eczema and dermatitis can also be exacerbated with the use of these products.

We have a great variety of ways in which you can make hand sanitizers at home. In order to avoid the adverse effects of these commercially produced hand sanitizers, and to ensure good health, it is essential to know some home made recipes too.

Types of hand sanitizer:

There are two main types of hand sanitizers that are available for use. These are:

- Alcohol based hand sanitizers

- Alcohol free hand sanitizers

It would not be wise to compare one with the other or try to prove which one is better amongst the two. It is important to know the differences between these types so that you know when to use what.

Alcohol based hand sanitizers are the most common variety of hand sanitizers used worldwide. It is also recommended by many health experts and healthcare organizations. The alcohol present in these sanitizers is the main ingredient that acts against the germs present on our hands. It helps in destroying the proteins in certain viruses and bacteria, rendering them harmless.

Non-alcohol based sanitizers use products like aloe vera or witch hazel instead of alcohol to provide the antimicrobial property. These are mainly used in people who have sensitivity for alcohol based products. It is also used in children in whom the use of products containing such large quantities of alcohol is not recommended. In the following chapter we not only discuss in detail about the main ingredients used in making these different kinds of sanitizers, we also talk about the recipes that you can use to make them at home.

Chapter 3:

Make your own Hand Sanitizer

With the advent of Covid-19 and its spread throughout the world, panic ensued. This led to people stockpiling goods and essentials and led to a shortage of many items in the market. This includes canned food, toilet papers, non-perishable food items. Another thing that has gone short in the markets following the spread of the pandemic is a hand sanitizer.

The news of impending disease led many people to stockpile goods and buy them in huge quantities. There are thousands of new brands of sanitizers that you might have never heard of before. This amassing of products also resulted in shortage of these items and eventually a hike in prices. A lot of people when looking for these products online find the prices to be hiked up to even five or ten folds. Thus, it makes it very difficult to even buy one bottle of a hand sanitizer during a crisis like this.

A hand sanitizer is simply a liquid or gel that helps in protection against microbes that cause illnesses. The main ingredient that achieves this purpose of decontamination is the different types of alcohol. It does so by denaturing the proteins present in viruses or bacteria.

But do we really need hand sanitizers when we could just go and wash your hands?

Well, the answer is yes. Even though it is true that handwashing is the first thing you should start practicing to reduce transmission of diseases, there are many instances in which you do not have access to soap and clean water. In these scenarios, a hand sanitizer will be a very important product to use to protect against germs.

Hand sanitizers in healthcare setting:

Another very important use of hand sanitizers is in a healthcare setting. CDC has outlined the guidelines for the use of hand sanitizers specifically for healthcare workers. According to these guidelines, it is important for healthcare workers to wash their hands with antibacterial soap and water to remove all the visible dirt or bodily fluids like blood and faeces. It is important to clean visible dirt because hand sanitizers are not useful if there is visible dirt on the hands. On the other hand, if the hands are visibly clean, all healthcare workers are recommended to use an alcohol based hand sanitizer for protection against the germs.These recommendation and guidelines have led to an increase in the use of hand sanitizers in the hospital settings. This does not apply only to doctors, but also to nurses or any other staff that is in contact with patients. Alcoholic hand sanitizers have a great log reduction of different kinds of bacteria like gram positive or gram negative bacteria, as well as certain fungi and viruses. It is still very important for healthcare professionals to use hand sanitizers in conjunction with practicing handwashing using antimicrobial soap and water too.

Hand sanitizers are essential in protecting yourself against many microorganisms that can pose a threat to your health. These products are available in bottles of different sizes and you can easily get a pocket friendly bottle from any departmental store or pharmacy. Hand sanitizers are also available in different forms. These include gels, sprays or foams. The most commonly used form is the gels. On the other hand, foams are usually very expensive and so they are least common. In addition to that, they are also available in different formulations and thick ones are preferred over the thin ones. Even though there is a huge variety of hand sanitizers available commercially, there are many ways in which you can make it at home and avoid all the hassle.

Making a hand sanitizer at home is not a complicated task. On the other hand, it is not as easy as it sounds either. But with the right guidance, you can easily try this at home too.

There are a few things that should be kept in mind before attempting to make your own hand sanitizer:

To make an effective formula, it is absolutely crucial that you use the same quantities and same concentrations as required. Changing the quantity or making imprecise measurements can lead to your formula being totally ineffective or even harmful. Therefore, the first step is to know the right ingredients, their quantities and to measure them accurately.

Use a clean counter top on which you are preparing this concoction. Preferably, you can clean the surface with diluted bleach to disinfect it first. Clean your own hands with soap and water. It is very important that the tools that you use for measurement while making sanitizer are sterilised or at least properly washed. WHO also recommends that after you have made your own sanitizer, you need to first let it sit for about 72 hours to allow the alcohol to kill any bacteria if present.

Do not use drinking alcohol if it is not at least 60% in

concentration. Lower concentrations will not allow the breakage of lipid layers of viruses in order to kill them or make them harmless. Make sure that you are using the right kind of alcohol. As a recommendation, 99% isopropyl alcohol (rubbing alcohol) or ethanol (grain alcohol, most commonly available at 90%-95%) should be used. Avoid using other types of alcohol (e.g., methanol), as they can be toxic.

A hand sanitizer can never be a complete substitute for hand washing.WHO recommends the adequate hand washing practices that are mentioned in Chapter 1 to be acquired to keep yourself safe from the germs. Now that you know what safety precautions to take, let's move on towards some recipes of these sanitizers that you can try making yourself.

A hand sanitizer has a large quantity of alcohol which is also the main ingredient. Make sure that it is kept away from heat and flame. The alcohol used in these products is highly flammable and can lead to accidents. Smoking or flames should not be allowed in the area where it is being prepared.

It is also important to note that it should be kept away from the reach of the children. Ingestion of large amounts can lead to toxicity. A healthcare provider should be immediately contacted in case there is an emergency. According to CDC, From 2011 – 2015, U.S. poison control centers received nearly 85,000 calls related to these accidents among children.

In this chapter, we will talk about the different ways in which we can make hand sanitizers at home.

First, let's discuss the main ingredients that are mostly required in making DIY hand sanitizers:

1. **Alcohol:** As mentioned previously, alcohol acts as the main ingredient to disinfect and kill microorganisms. The most important quality of the alcohol used in these formulations is its concentration. Rubbing alcohol, or isopropyl alcohol is the recommended one. It is a colorless chemical with a very strong smell. Note that it is also highly flammable, so it needs to be handled with care. It has many industrial and pharmaceutical uses. It is able to dissolve a wide range of compounds and so is commonly used as a solvent. It can be used for cleaning in optometry or electronics. It can also be used as a preservative in medical sciences or in disinfecting pads. It is mostly combined with water when using it in a

hand sanitizer. A 75% v/v solution in water is frequently used. Keep in mind that ingestion or inhalation of large quantities can lead to toxicity. The most common symptoms of toxicity include nausea, vomiting, dizziness, headache, respiratory depression or coma. Ethanol is another alcohol that is also used in some hand sanitizers. It is also called grain alcohol or drinking alcohol. It is produced by sugar fermentation and is also volatile and flammable. This is the type of alcohol that we use in drinks. Ethanol can be used as fuel or as a solvent. In medical setups, it is used as a disinfectant in wipes, pads or sanitizers. Although it is ineffective against the spores of bacteria, it usually kills them by destroying their proteins. It also disturbs the osmotic pressure of the cells leading to its dehydration and shrinkage and eventually death. This warrants its use as an antiseptic.

2. **Aloe Vera:** An evergreen succulent plant of genus Aloe, Aloe Vera is usually grown in hot and arid climates like the tropics. It has plenty of uses , for example, as an ornamental plant, in cosmetics as well as in medicine. Aloe vera has a clear gel and a latex that can be used for different purposes

Aloe Vera gel is one of the most commonly used products in skincare. It can be used to treat acne, burns, rash or dry skin. Aloe vera provides a soothing effect to dry skin and hydrates it. That is why it is also an important ingredient that can be used in the making of hand sanitizers to keep the skin fresh. One of the most commonly used herbal remedies for skin, Aloe vera gel can be extracted directly from its leaves too. You can break the leaf apart and press out the gel ready for use. You can also get commercially available Aloe vera gel if you don't have access to the plant. It is important to note, however, that Aloe vera can be irritating in some skin conditions too and you may experience itching sensation after use. It is important to apply a small quantity first to make sure that your skin is not reacting adversely to it. Do not take Aloe vera orally and keep it out of the reach of children. The main use of Aloe vera gel in hand sanitizers is its moisturizing effect on the skin. You might have heard a common complaint that hand sanitizers leave your hands irritable. This is because when the high amount of alcohol in these products dries off, it leaves the skin dry and prone to sensitivity. This is where Aloe vera comes in. Hand sanitizers with added Aloe vera helps in leaving a protective moisturizing layer on your hands after use. This makes your skin smooth and soft.

3. **Hydrogen peroxide:** This is another common ingredient used mostly in sanitizing sprays. Hydrogen peroxide is readily available everywhere for a very small amount. It can be mixed with a little water to make it last for a longer time. The reason behind adding a little quantity of hydrogen peroxide is to kill the bacterial spores that might contaminate the solution. Low concentrations are used as it is highly corrosive in higher concentrations.

4. **Glycerol:** Glycerol, also called glycerin, is another ingredient that can be used in sanitizers to keep the skin moisturised. Similar to Aloe vera, this also helps in preventing drying out of hands after use. It is called a humectant. A humectant is a substance used to retain moisture. It is often a molecule with several hydrophilic, that is water loving, groups. It is safe to use and cheaply available in local stores. It also has antimicrobial and antiviral properties. It is gentle on the skin and can be used in people who have sensitive skin. It

should be noted that using a higher percentage of glycerin may add to the stickiness of the solution.

5. **Essential Oils:** There is no harm in making your hand sanitizer smell good. Essential oils are fragrances of plants used in perfumes, soaps or incense. It is important to note that essential oils can be irritating to some skins. They are also dangerous if used in large quantities as they can be toxic. Some say that essential oils produce a healing and calming effect. This is why it is mostly used for aromatherapy too. We also add a bit of essential oils in hand sanitizers to make them smell nice and have these healing effects on the skin. Although it is worth mentioning that WHO does not recommend adding any fragrances as it might lead to an allergic reaction.

6. **Water:** It is advisable to use boiled or distilled water to make sure that it is free of germs. Normally, water is used at room temperature. Just make sure that there are no visible particles in the water that is being used.

Now we will talk about a number of recipes that you can follow to make your own hand sanitizer at home and you can choose the ones that suit you the best.

Alcoholic hand sanitizer recipes

- **The Emergency Recipe**

First, we'll talk about the most basic gel recipe that you can use to formulate your sanitizer quickly and efficiently at home.

What you need:

1. Isopropyl alcohol (99 percent preferably)
2. Aloe vera gel
3. Small bottle

How to make it:

This is the most basic recipe and all you have to do is mix 3 parts alcohol with 1 part of aloe vera gel. Use a small bottle and pour the mixture in it. Let it sit for some time before using it.

- **A Large Batch:**

WHO has provided guidelines on how to prepare a huge batch of sanitizer for community use. Keep in mind that this is for large-scale production of sanitizer and such large quantities might not be needed for individual use..

For a general idea, a list of ingredients used in the large scale production, as outlined by the WHO is also provided as follows.

What you need:

1. 96% ethanol or 99.8% isopropyl alcohol

2. 98% glycerin

3. 3% hydrogen peroxide

4. Distilled or boiled water

5. Plastic bottles, measuring cylinders

6. An alcoholometer: It has temperature at the bottom and percentage of ethanol at the top. An alcoholometer is used in commercial production to make sure that the correct concentration of alcohol is being used while preparing the formulation. This maintains the accuracy and keeps the sanitizer effective. It can also be used at the end to confirm that the required concentration of alcohol is present. Any percentage below the required percentage can render the sanitizer useless.

The following formulation is recommended by WHO for a 10 Litre preparation:

1. Ethanol: 8333 ml

2. Glycerin: 145 ml

3. Hydrogen peroxide: 417 ml

Note: Use the same concentrations as mentioned above.

How to make it:

1. Alcohol is poured into a large, graduated bottle, using a funnel if needed.

2. Using a measuring cylinder, required amounts of hydrogen peroxide and glycerol are added. Make sure to rinse the measuring cylinder with distilled water as the viscous glycerin sticks to the walls of the container it is poured in.

3. The bottle is then filled with water upto the 10 litre mark to finalise the preparation.

4. The bottle is capped and the solution is mixed by gently shaking the bottle.

5. Now that the sanitizer is ready, it is split up into

as many small bottles as required. Make sure that 72 hours are given before use of this solution. This time allows the alcohol in the solution to kill any bacteria that might have contaminated it during the preparation.

The final concentrations of the constituents in this sanitizer are as follows:

1. Ethanol: 80% (v/v)

2. Glycerol: 1.45% (v/v)

3. Hydrogen peroxide: 0.125% (v/v)

- **The Spray Recipe**

Another way to use a hand sanitizer is to use it in the spray form. This is a recipe provided on WIRED to produce a small quantity of this disinfectant spray.

What you need:

1. Isopropyl alcohol: 1 ⅔ cups

2. Glycerin: 2 teaspoons

3. Hydrogen peroxide: 1 tablespoon

4. Distilled water as required

5. A spray bottle

How to make it:

In a clean container, pour the given amount of alcohol. Add 2 teaspoons of glycerin in it. This will make sure that your hands are not left dry after using the sanitizer. Then add hydrogen peroxide. You can now add about ¼ cups of distilled water and your solution is ready.

This solution can be transferred into a spray bottle and used as needed. It can be used as a disinfectant on table tops or other surfaces too as the spray form makes it easier to use it that way.

- **A mix of natural products**

One of our most favorite recipes is this hand sanitizer that requires comparatively more ingredients but makes for an effective antimicrobial. This is also different in no a way that this is stronger than many all natural handmade hand sanitizers. Let's learn how to make this.

What you need:

1. Essential oils of your choice

2. Rubbing alcohol

3. Glycerin

4. Aloe vera

5. Distilled water

6. Germ destroyer oil

How to make it:

¼ cup of aloe vera gel is added into a container of choice. To this, add 1 tablespoon rubbing alcohol after checking its concentration. The rubbing alcohol used should be at least 60% in concentration as recommended by experts. Glycerin can also be added to change the consistency. Adding too much glycerin can make it sticky.

A few drops of a variety of essential oils of your choice are now added. More commonly used essential oils are tea tree oil, peppermint oil, lemongrass oil.

A small quantity of distilled water is added according to the consistency that you require. Germ destroyer essential oil can also be added to this to increase its effectiveness.

This mixture is now added in a small bottle and left for a few hours to settle.

Your sanitizer is ready to use.

Non-Alcoholic hand sanitizer recipes

Alcoholic hand sanitizers are available everywhere in the market. But some people want to use the non alcoholic versions too.This is due to the fact that some alcoholic sanitizers can be very irritating on the skin. Another common reason is that it is not advisable to use hand sanitizers on children. Using sanitizers with high alcohol content can be very damaging to the skin of children. It can not only dry the skin excessively, but it also has the potential to have adverse reactions on the skin. If we talk about baby skin in particular, it is worth keeping in mind that their skin is very sensitive and prone to damage by chemicals.

We have compiled some non alcoholic hand sanitizers that can be used in such cases. Many of these recipes have ingredients that are easily available in every kitchen. Therefore, it can also be used in cases of emergency or shortage.

Let's talk about some of the common recipes that people have been using to keep their hands clean and germ free.

- **White Vinegar:**

You must have heard about this one before! Acetic acid, also known as white vinegar, is an inexpensive disinfectant that has been used for many years. The best thing about vinegar is that it is not only biodegradable but it does not have the potential to cause toxicity as some commercially available alcoholic sanitizers might. In a study conducted in the UK on the effectiveness of household agents against the flu virus, it was seen that 10% malt vinegar proved to be really effective against these viruses. It works by inactivating the virus making it harmless.

The normal concentration that is available in local stores is usually 5% white vinegar. In some studies, it is mentioned to be more than 70% effective against all kinds of germs. It can be used as it is, or diluted with water if full strength is not required.

But how does it work? Like other disinfectants, vinegar also works by damaging the protein machinery of the cells of these germs rendering them harmless.

How to use it?

It is recommended to use white vinegar diluted with water in 50/50 ratio. An easy way is to add equal quantities of both in a spray bottle and use it on the go. It can be used on table tops, kitchen counters, walls and windows or any other surface that is frequently touched. As a hand sanitizer, white vinegar can be added in a small spray bottle and sprayed all over the hands whenever needed.

Are other forms of vinegar as effective as white vinegar? At many places, apple cider vinegar is also mentioned as a disinfectant. It is, however, worth mentioning that these other varieties of vinegar are seen to be less effective and weaker than white vinegar.

Should we use vinegar as a substitute for commercial cleaning products?

Although vinegar can be used as a disinfectant in a variety of settings, but in places where a very strong sanitizer is needed, it is recommended to use another stronger disinfectant.

What kind of bacteria can it kill? It is commonly seen to be effective against Salmonella, E. Coli, tuberculosis, among others.

Will it be effective against the Covid-19? Well, there is no evidence to prove how effective white vinegar can be against Corona virus. The Covid-19 variety is a recently discovered one, therefore, scientists are still trying to find out the properties of this virus. It is, however, seen in many studies that white vinegar is more effective against bacteria than it is against some viruses.

What if you cannot tolerate the strong smell of vinegar?

There is a way around this problem too. Even though vinegar evaporates and does not leave much odor after some time, but if people are concerned about this smell, a few drops of any essential oil can be added. This includes tea tree or eucalyptus.

Note: Do not combine vinegar with bleach or hydrogen peroxide.

- **Tea tree oil:**

A question that arises in everybody's mind is, what exactly is tea tree oil and why is it used as a remedy for so many things?

Well, we are here to answer these queries.

Tea tree oil is also known as melaleuca oil. As the name suggests, this oil is derived from the leaves of tea tree that is found mainly in the UK and Australia. This oil is used for a plenty of skin conditions including acne and fungal infections. It is also seen in many cases, however, that tea tree oil can be irritating to the skin and may cause allergic reactions. Before using it, a small quantity can be applied on a part of skin to see if it is producing any allergic reaction. A small quantity of vitamin E can also be added in the solution to make it less irritating.

How to use it? Take a small bottle and add four ounces of distilled water in it. Now, ten drops of tea tree oil can be added in this water to make a disinfectant solution. This can be used in the form of a spray.

There is another recipe that can also be used to make hand sanitizer using tea tree oil. For this recipe, take 6 ounces of distilled water and add ten drops of essential oil (tea tree oil) as mentioned previously. Now add 1 teaspoon of castile soap in this concoction. We will give a small introduction of castile soap for those who are not aware of it:

Castile soap is a soap made from olive oil, coconut oil or any other plant based oil. It gets its name Castile from a historical region in Spain. Castile soaps have a very long history and these hard soaps are said to be made as early as the 11th century, according to some historians.

The purpose of adding castile soap in our sanitizer is that

it can help in dissolving the oils. It also acts as a surfactant. The good news is that castile soap is biodegradable and non-toxic too.

How does it work? Tea tree oil does not only work against viruses, bacteria or fungi, but it also provides anti inflammatory properties, as some studies have mentioned.

It should be noted that tea tree oil is not safe to be consumed orally. Therefore, it is absolutely essential that it is kept away from the reach of children and not used around the mouth.

- **Foaming hand sanitizer:**

Another very commonly used recipe for hand sanitizers is a foaming hand sanitizer recipe. It is a simple and easy to follow recipe that can be completed in a few minutes in total.

What you need:

1. Foaming container: It is absolutely essential to get a foaming container because this is exactly what makes this a foaming cleanser. It is also called a foam pump or a squeezer and can be easily ordered online too. It simply emits the liquid in

the bottle in the form of a foam. Some people tend to prefer this to gels or liquids.

2. Witch Hazel

3. Aloe vera

4. Tea tree oil or any other essential oil for fragrance.

How to make it:

3 tablespoons of aloe vera gel are combined with one tablespoon of witch hazel. To this, your own choice of essential oils can be added. The one most commonly mentioned is Young Living Thieves essential oil. Make sure that you are not using too much essential oils as it can cause irritation or breakouts.

All of these ingredients are mixed and transferred to a foaming container. Your natural hand sanitizer is ready for use.

Another recipe is also available for making foaming hand sanitizer. It uses mostly the same ingredients with little changes.

What you need:

- Castile soap
- Essential Oils
- Distilled water

How to make it:

Half a teaspoon of castile soap is added into the foaming container (a small bottle, standard size). To this a few drops of essential oils of your choice (a combination of two or three) are added. This mixture is mixed and water is poured to fill the container. Do not add too much water.

- **Hydrogen peroxide**

Hydrogen peroxide is a strong chemical that can be directly used as a disinfectant too. It decomposes easily into water and oxygen. This is a very simple and straightforward recipe that can be used when disinfection is required. Hydrogen peroxide is said to be effective against a wide variety of bacteria and viruses. Many health experts have said that we can use hydrogen peroxide and some other strong household agents to disinfect our houses from viruses like Corona too. However, the evidence still remains unreliable.

What you need:

1. A 3% hydrogen peroxide variety is available most commonly for use

2. A small, dark container is needed because when exposed to light, hydrogen peroxide can be easily oxidized making it useless.

How to make it:

A 3% solution of hydrogen peroxide is added to a dark container. Usually a small spray bottle can be handy to use. Another option is to use a foam pump. Either way, it should cover both hands adequately. Just like the other hand sanitizers, you can rub your hands until it becomes dry. You can also dilute it with a little water.

- **Eucalyptus**

Eucalyptus is an evergreen tree that has been used for a very long time for its health related properties. The oil from these trees is commonly used in flavorings or perfumes, and also as an antibacterial. The oil has a very strong woody scent. The oil also has antioxidant and anti-inflammatory properties.

It is interesting to note that in the 19th century, oil extracted from these trees was used to clean urinary catheters in the hospitals. These antimicrobial properties have also been used in making dental mouthwashes from eucalyptus oil.

We also have a recipe for a had sanitizer that takes advantage of the antimicrobial properties of eucalyptus

What you need:

- Eucalyptus oil and any other essential oil
- Aloe vera gel or liquid
- Distilled water
- Small container
- Vitamin E serum (optional)

How to make it:

Take a small container and add 2 ounces of Aloe vera gel or juice (according to the consistency required).

To this, add 15 drops of eucalyptus and 5 drops of any other essential oil of choice.

You can also add a small quantity of vitamin E to keep your hands moisturized.

- **Witch Hazel:**

Witch hazel is quite an interesting name for a plant, don't you think? Well, the word 'witch' in this name comes from an old English word wiche, which means bendable. It is a deciduous shrub found in North America, Japan and China. In North America, it is also referred to as 'winterbloom'.

Witch hazel has been used in medicine for a very long time. Its extract mostly consists of gallotannins and safrole among other things. It can be found in medical stores by the name of witch hazel water. It is also used in the form of gel or cream in patients that have skin irritation. It also retains moisture and prevents dryness and eczema in some people. The gallic acid and tannins present in this plant are anti-inflammatory agents that can help soothe inflammatory conditions including some conditions of the skin.

A very interesting thing to note, however, is that witch hazel is also an antimicrobial- in particular an antiviral. The question is, what quality of a witch hazel plant renders it useful against the viruses?

Some test tube studies conducted in the past have shown witch hazel to be effective against some viruses like

Herpes Simplex. Research conducted showed that the tannins in the witch hazel plant, particularly the Hamamelis virginiana species, impart these plants potent activity against certain viruses. The extract has also shown to be effective against Influenza virus.

Witch hazel is not seen to be dangerous when applied topically. It can be used safely several times a day as per the requirement and helps in soothing of the skin. In some people with sensitive skin, however, it can cause allergy. Therefore, before using it extensively it is safe to apply a small amount on a part of the skin to see if it produces any adverse reaction. It should be noted that it is not recommended to take witch hazel water orally as it might prove toxic.

There are quite a few recipes in which hazel witch plant extract can be used as a hand sanitizer. We will start with the most basic recipe that you can follow to make this kind of hand sanitizer at home.

What you need:

1. Witch Hazel

2. Aloe vera juice

3. Essential oils

How to make it:

For this recipe, you need to add 1 cup of aloe vera juice in a small container. Make sure all the tools that you are using are clean, including your hands.

Pour 1/2 cup of witch hazel in the aloe vera juice.

Now, around 10 drops of essential oils can be added in this mixture. The oils you can use are tea tree, eucalyptus, or cinnamon.

Blend the mixture well and keep it in an airtight container.

Keep this mixture away from direct sunlight.

Another recipe with witch hazel extract can also be used. This has some more ingredients added to it in case you have these easily available.

What you need:

- Witch Hazel
- Aloe vera
- Distilled water
- Essential oil

- Vitamin E oil
- Spray bottle

How to make it:

In a small container, add 3 tablespoons of witch hazel and aloe vera and mix it well.

Now add ten drops of tea tree oil and ten drops of eucalyptus oil in this mixture.

Adding vitamin E oil is optional but it helps with retaining moisture.

Transfer this mixture to a 20 ounce spray bottle and shake it well.

- **Coconut oil'**

Coconut oil has been a very popular product that is widely used in treatment of many skin and hair conditions. It is a highly saturated oil extracted from the raw coconuts, and is solid at room temperature. It has a large quantity of saturated medium chain fatty acids. These acids give this oil the antimicrobial property that it is well known for, especially the lauric acid. Like witch hazel, test tube studies have also been conducted on coconut oil and proved it to be effective against many microbes. It also reduces inflammation and has antioxidants in it. Another important property of coconut oil is that it is moisturizing and can be used for the treatment or prevention of dry skin.

Keeping in view its hydrating and antimicrobial properties, we have recipes that use coconut oil as an important ingredient too.

What you need:

1. Coconut oil

2. Aloe vera juice

3. Vitamin E oil

How to make it:

Pour 3 tablespoons of aloe vera in a small bottle. Add around 1 teaspoon of fractionated coconut oil that is readily available at stores. You can add a ½ teaspoon of vitamin E oil in this mixture. Vitamin E is well known for its beneficial effects on skin. To add a little fragrance to it and make it smell nice, you can add a few drops of essential oils like tea tree or peppermint in this mixture.

Use a spray bottle for this hand sanitizer and store it in a cool, dry place.

Hand sanitizer for kids:

We all know how sensitive the skin of kids is. You wouldn't want to irritate this baby skin and for that it is important to minimize the use of chemicals. Hand sanitizers that are commercially available may contain agents that can prove to be harsh for children. Alcohol also can lead to dryness and itching. WELLNESSMAMA has provided an amazing recipe for hand sanitizers that can be used especially for kids. The best part about this recipe is that it is made from all natural products, which means that you don't need to worry about those nasty chemicals getting on your kids' hands. So let's get on with it.

What you need:

- Aloe vera gel
- Essential oil

How to make it:

Take ¼ cup of aloe vera gel in a small container. This can be purchased from any local store. It can also be directly taken out by pressing the aloe vera leaves.

Add about 20 drops of essential oils of your choice in the gel.

Mix the solution properly and transfer it to a small bottle or a silicone tube.

Store in a cool, dry place.

We also have another elaborate hand sanitizer recipe that is safe for kids too. This one uses coconut oil as well as geranium and lavender oils. We have already discussed the efficacy of coconut oil, so let's move on and talk about the other two essential oils that we will be using in this recipe

Geranium oil:

Geranium essential oil is extracted from the leaves of Pelargonium graveolens. It is an uncommon species of plant present in the regions of South Africa and Zimbabwe. These plants are very strong scented and are used in perfumes and cosmetics. Like other essential oils, geranium oil is also believed to have antibacterial, antiviral and astringent properties. It is known to provide a soothing effect on the skin and is used in skin conditions like eczema or psoriasis. It also has anti-inflammatory properties that make it effective against these skin problems.

A study conducted on the effectiveness of these species found that geranium essential oil was as effective as certain antibiotics in warding off bacteria like Staphylococcus Aureus, present commonly on the skin. It also helps in reducing itching from allergic reactions.

The reason we are using geranium oil in our recipe is because it is safe for babies aged 6 months and above and can be safely used in making hand sanitizers for kids.

Lavender oil:

This essential oil is obtained by steam distillation from lavender flowers. It has two different forms, lavender oil and lavender spike oil. And has a nice smell. Lavender oil has been widely used to treat acne. Its antiinflammatory properties help in making it an effective therapy against acne breakouts or eczematous skin. It can also be used as a facial toner when mixed with hazel witch water. It is seen to have skin healing properties too. Owing to all of these beneficial effects on skin and the fact that these are safe for young babies, we are using lavender oil in the following recipe.

What you need:

1. Coconut oil

2. Aloe vera gel

3. Geranium oil

4. Lavender oil

5. Witch Hazel

How to make it:

First, you need to take 1 tablespoon of melted coconut oil. Since coconut oil is solid at room temperature, you will need to heat it first.

Now add ¼ cup of aloe vera gel and mix the two well.

When the coconut oil and aloe vera gel have mixed together, add 1 ½ tablespoon of witch hazel water to it.

Now add 5 drops each of both lavender oil and geranium oil.

Transfer it into a small plastic or glass bottle.

Your hand sanitizer is ready for use.

We also wanted to include some recipes of antibacterial soaps and wipes to aid you in maintaining hand hygiene. So, let's go on and see how to make our own antibacterial soap.

What you need:

1. Castile soap
2. Distilled water
3. Almond oil
4. Glycerin
5. Essential oil

How to make it:

In a container, add some castile soap. Now add 1 tablespoon of glycerin and 2 tablespoon of almond oil in it.

You have an option of adding the essential oils of your own choice. Some recommendations include tea tree oil, eucalyptus, lavander.

Fill the rest of the bottle with distilled water and mix it well. Your anti-bacterial hand soap is ready for use.

A simple recipe of making wipes is as follows:

What you need:

1. Individual paper towels
2. White vinegar
3. Distilled water
4. Dish detergent
5. Essential oil

How to make it:

Take one cup white vinegar in a clean, plastic container and add one cup of water in it. Now add a few drops of liquid detergent and your own choice of essential oil for fragrance.

Place the paper towels in the container in which you have to keep the wipes.

Pour all the combined ingredients over the paper towels in the container. Make sure the wipes are soaked in this liquid.

Store in a cool, dry place.

Chapter 4:

Safety Consideration

Leading a healthy life is and should be the top most priority for every person. Being on a sick bed makes us realize how lucky being healthy is, and how grateful we should be for every moment we spend disease free.

The world that we are living in today is becoming increasingly dangerous. The reason is not just the political turmoil that every country is in, but also the increasing rate of natural calamities that we are facing.

With the start of the year 2020, we saw the world changing before our very eyes. Climate change was the real threat following us for the last few years, the fear of losing our planet to increasingly hazardous effects of carbon emissions.

If this wasn't enough, Coronavirus pandemic hit us like it has never before. Considered and called out for being 'just a flu' for the first few days that it emerged, this disease changed its course and took everyone by surprise. Starting from China, it spread on to become a global pandemic, engulfing giant countries like the US. In the midst of all the panic that ensued following the spread of Covid-19, human kind suffered from crisis after crisis. From shortage of toilet papers and hand sanitizers to basic food necessities, we saw it all.

When it became increasingly clear that the shortage of these hygiene products was inevitable and the hikes in their prices in some countries made it impossible for a common man to buy them, we turned to something else. We started trying to make soaps and hand sanitizers at home. This book also aims at helping you with the very same thing. It is very important to be calm and not panic while we fight together with these viruses that are attacking us so frequently.

There are some healthcare safety tips that we have combined here to help you stay safe from a very large number of diseases. These are simple yet effective strategies to stay safe from the dangers that we are facing these days.

How to prevent yourself from getting sick:

1. **Keep your hands clean**

Wash, wash and wash

This has been our mantra from the very start. No matter what else you do to keep yourself safe from disease, do not forget that handwashing should be your number one priority. Handwashing alone can help save you from many illnesses. Our hands consciously and unconsciously get in contact with many contaminated surfaces throughout the day, and when these hands touch the mucus membranes of the body, bacteria and viruses get a free pass inside you.

If you do not have access to clean water and soap everywhere, an alcohol based hand sanitizer can be your next best friend. Check out our recipes for homemade alcohol based hand sanitizers in the previous chapter, if you haven't already. Washing hands can literally save lives.

2. Stay at home when you are sick

Another important thing to keep in mind is that there are countless contagious diseases, even a simple cold or flu, that can spread if you go out unnecessarily while you are sick. Even in the pandemic like Covid-19, the best advice that the health experts gave was to self isolate in case you feel sick. By staying at home, you can prevent spreading illnesses to other people. In the recent Covid-19 scenario, using health measures and self-quarantine itself helped a lot and kept the hospitals from getting overwhelmingly full.

3. Eat green vegetables

A lot of people don't like eating vegetables, especially the boring greens. Well, this time you should keep in mind that the green vegetables are full of nutritious juices and a wide variety of vitamins. Taking plenty of vitamins can help keep you away from many diseases. It fortifies your immune system and helps you in fighting viral infections specifically.

4. Get proper sleep

We cannot stress more on how important sleep is to keep your body healthy and fit. Sleep essentially restores your body and makes you a new person every morning you wake up. Sleep replenishes your body and reinvigorates it. Another important thing to keep in mind is that an adequate amount of sleep helps you in fighting off microbes and helps in building resistance against viral attacks.

5. Get vaccinated!

Remember that the only thing that is going to save you from many fatal diseases is a dose of vaccine. Vaccine does not damage your body, and no, it does not give you more diseases. In simple words, it is merely a harmless form of microbes that is injected into your body so that the body can recognize it and build immunity. So, the next time that microbe attacks, your body will already know how to fight against it and will not be taken by surprise.

6. Take proper nutrition

Your body is going to build from the food you eat. If you eat healthy, your mind and body stays healthy, and if you don't, you get sick. There are many foods that can specifically help in building your immunity. We have made a list of a few foods to get you started:

- Citrus fruits: Citrus fruits contain a large amount of vitamin C. Vitamin C is our saviour in fighting against diseases, specifically viral illness. It helps in building your immunity by increasing the number of white blood cells in the body. These include lemons, oranges, grapefruit.

- Spinach: Ever wondered why the health experts always advise you to eat green veggies like spinach regularly? It is because spinach is a wonderous vegetable. It is not only rich in vitamin C but also provides your body with a wide variety of antioxidants to keep you healthy

- Sunflower seeds: Not widely eaten, but sunflower seeds are packed with nutrients. The most important nutrient in these seeds is Vitamin E. Like vitamin C, vitamin E also helps to some extent in building your immunity. Vitamin E also acts as an antioxidant.

Now that we have briefly discussed how some important safety measures can help you stay away from diseases, let's get back to hand hygiene as it is the single most important factor in prevention of illnesses.

Hand sanitizers play a very important part in maintenance of hygiene. Water and soap are not accessible everywhere and that is why hand sanitizers can help ward off bacterias and viruses for some time. Like every other product, the efficacy of hand sanitizers also depend on its adequate usage. It is very important to know how to properly use these products and what safety concerns should be kept in mind while using them

We have already discussed the dangers posed by

commercially produced hand sanitizers in Chapter 2. Here we will give you a quick summary on what to avoid and keep in mind while using hand sanitizers, whether commercially produced or handmade.

What to keep in mind while using hand sanitizers:

- Hand sanitizers, while being very important for hygiene, do not substitute hand washing. These cannot be used on your hands if there is visible dirt on it. In these cases, you must wash your hands first to remove the dirt.

- It is important to know the composition of the products that you are using. Products that contain large quantities of chemicals will do more harm than good.

- Make sure that you are not using a large quantity of essential oils in your homemade preparations. Although essential oils give a soothing effect to the skin, excessive use is not advised.

- Try to test a small quantity of whichever product you use on a small patch of skin first. Every person's skin is different and while one product is suitable for one skin, it might not be good for another person. In people that have sensitive skin type, using harsh chemicals or excessive drying of skin produces adverse reactions and may cause damage. It is important to report to a healthcare professional if you are having any serious symptoms

- Keep these products out of the reach of children as many of them might contain ingredients that can be toxic if ingested orally. When you make hand sanitizers at home and do not label them or keep them away from the kids, there is a chance of accidental ingestion that might prove hazardous. In case it does happen, it is advisable to take the child directly to the emergency room and inform them timely.

Illnesses like coronavirus or influenza have been seen to wreak havoc all across the world. An important thing to keep in mind is not to panic while the whole world is doing so. In this book, we managed to educate you not only about the basics of hand sanitizer usage but also on the pros and cons and safety measures to take while using them. The wide variety of recipes, provided in chapter 3, can help in saving you from all the trouble and help you in making hand sanitizers at home. Remember, prevention is better than cure and together we can fight against any calamities that may befall.